Nourishing Your Newborn

A Commonsense Guide for Those First Few Days

by **Carolyn K. Gilmore**, RNC-E

Registered Nurse, Certified in Obstetrics, Retired

"These methods aren't always conventional, nor are they taught in books. They come from years of personal experience—and they work!"

Independently published by
Carolyn K. Gilmore

Nourishing Your Newborn:
A Commonsense Guide for Those First Few Days
©Copyright 2012, Carolyn K. Gilmore, RNC-E

Written and Illustrated by Carolyn K. Gilmore
Webeii@aol.com

ISBN 978-0-9850209-0-3

DISCLAIMER:
Every effort has been made on the part of the author to provide accurate and helpful information based on years of clinical experience. However, the author assumes no responsibility for outcomes related to the application of the contents of this booklet. If questions remain about breastfeeding that this booklet does not cover, mothers should seek medical advice from their primary care provider or the baby's pediatrician.

Edited by Chris Nordquist
The Write Stuff
Dundee, Oregon

Printed in the United States of America

Layout and design
Gail Watson

Additional copies of this book can be purchased at:
www.createspace.com/3770364

Dedication

*This book is dedicated to nursing mothers
and their babies everywhere.*

"In my 41 years as an obstetrics nurse, I learned
a variety of ways to teach both mother
and baby how to succeed at breastfeeding. These
methods ("tidbits") aren't always conventional, nor
are they taught in books. They come from years of
personal experience—and they work!"

*Carolyn K. Gilmore, RNC-E
Registered Nurse, Certified in Obstetrics, Retired*

Contents

                                                                   Page
Introduction. i

SECTION I
Common Difficulties Encountered When Breastfeeding

CHAPTER 1   Nursing in the "Womb". 1

CHAPTER 2   Reasons Why Newborns May Have
             Difficulty (or Reluctance) Nursing 3

CHAPTER 3   Reasons Why Mothers May Contribute
             to Nursing Difficulties 13

SECTION II
Breastfeeding Solutions

CHAPTER 4   Properly Burping a Newborn & Other Helpful Tidbits 21

CHAPTER 5   Breastfeeding Positions. 23

CHAPTER 6   The Football Position. 25

CHAPTER 7   The Cross-Cuddle Position 31

CHAPTER 8   The Side-Lying Position 35

CHAPTER 9   Breast Care 43

SECTION III
When All Else Fails

CHAPTER 10   Nipple Confusion Versus Fluid Confusion 47

CHAPTER 11   **Special Needs Infants** 53
CHAPTER 12   **How Artificial Nipples Can Help** 57

Conclusion 63

Afterward 65

About the Author 69

Introduction

Why is it, if breastfeeding is such a "natural" act, so few mothers come home from the hospital successfully nursing their newborns? While everyone agrees that "mother's milk" is the best natural nourishment for newborns, breastfeeding does not always *feel* natural at first—either for the mother or her baby. One of the most common statements I heard in my 41 years as a neonatal nurse was, "My baby nursed so well the first time, but now he[1] just doesn't seem interested."

Too often, and especially after a successful first nursing experience, the mother assumes her baby will continue breastfeeding in the same way. Commonly, though, it is just the opposite. The newborn will either cry and not suck or he will be sleepy and disinterested. When this occurs, mothers begin to worry. Sometimes they even give up trying to nurse because the task becomes so daunting. Others return to the hospital days after delivery in order to meet with special "lactation consultants."

Serving mothers and newborns as an R.N.C. in obstetrics for most of my adult life, I assisted in approximately 2,200 deliveries

---

[1] **Note:** For the sake of readability, I have chosen to use the male pronoun (he, him, his) whenever referring to the newborn. Although I strongly support gender neutral language and (of course!) realize babies are born equally male and female, I found it easier to differentiate between mother (her) and baby (him) than to risk the kind of "she-her" confusion that results when talking about a mother and her female newborn.

and took care of nearly 17,000 newborns. I know just a little about breastfeeding! My concern through the years—and why I've decided to write this booklet—is the increasing number of mothers who simply give up nursing their newborns when faced with these *not-so-natural-feeling* challenges, and then feel like failed mothers as a result. I've lost track of the number of times I've run into mothers I've assisted, years after their deliveries, only to have them exclaim, "If it hadn't been for you, I would have bottle-fed my baby!"

Despite the large number of books, classes, and videos now available to guide young mothers in breastfeeding, I have found that these resources often fail to help. They rely largely on photographs and/or diagrams of older babies who have already established nursing patterns. For instance, many guides will show or suggest holding the baby in the cradle position (the most commonly known and "traditional" position for nursing). But this position is extremely difficult for most newborns to achieve, and, when their infants aren't able to latch on to the nipple or sustain sucking while cuddled this way, many mothers grow alarmed—a response that then creates its own set of problems.

Exasperated and discouraged mothers became my specialty over the years. I discovered that there are distinct reasons why a newborn seems disinterested in nursing after his first suckle, and I learned a variety of ways to teach both mother and baby how to succeed at breastfeeding. These methods ("tidbits") aren't always conventional, nor are they taught in books. They come from years of personal experience—and they work.

Common Difficulties Encountered When Breastfeeding

This section will explore the various factors contributing to why breastfeeding may feel so "difficult" for some mothers and infants. Problems may arise for *either* the newborn or mother, and many times these small impediments can combine to make breastfeeding feel less than pleasurable or satisfying. Later I will explore how to resolve these issues or avoid them altogether.

CHAPTER 1

"Nursing" in the Womb

One of the first things I tell a young mother when breastfeeding doesn't go according to plan is that she shouldn't worry: "*You* might have gone to class, but your baby didn't!" Her baby's resistance or apparent lack of interest in nursing is perfectly normal, even "natural." This is because a baby has been nursing (i.e., sucking and swallowing) without effort in the womb for the last several months. He has enjoyed a variety of nipples during that time, including fingers, thumbs, knees, lips, toes, and even his own tongue.

We've doubtless all heard the pun regarding "womb service." Well, it's true! In fact, a fetus never has to open his mouth much—or even actively suck—in order to obtain liquid. From the time he is 12 weeks old he has been increasing his fluid intake until he's averaging up to three glasses of amniotic fluid per day at the time of delivery—in addition to what he receives through the umbilical cord. The fluid rushes in automatically, without him even having to suck.

Consequently, when a baby finally makes his journey out of the womb, he has fully formed habits that take about 2 weeks to break. These habits include (1) not having to open his mouth wide to receive nourishment—let alone "latch on" and create suction, (2) not having

> "You might have gone to class, but your baby didn't!"
>
> "A baby's resistance or apparent lack of interest in nursing is perfectly normal, even 'natural.'"

1

been required to suck at a sustained rhythm to get the fluid he wanted or needed, and (3) sucking on a variety of slippery nipples that feel far different in shape and texture than the one his mother will present to him.[2] Likewise, he has grown used to being carried everywhere and feeling securely "encased" in a soft, warm, and moist environment.

Because a baby's sucking reflex is largely prompted by moisture on the inside of his mouth, a newborn is likely to nurse vigorously the first time he is put to his mother's nipple—even in the cradle position. His mouth is still moist from the amniotic fluid. Also, the stress of delivery can stimulate the sucking reflex. Consequently, when a healthy newborn nurses for the first time, everything feels "natural." The baby suckles contentedly, and the mother is relieved that he is safely in her arms at last.

That is why it is so surprising (and frustrating!) when the same baby acts as though he has never nursed before when he is returned to the nipple for subsequent feedings.

There are a variety of reasons why this may be so, which I will take time to examine here. First, I will look at this dilemma from the baby's perspective, to see why he may have difficulty and/or reluctance nursing. Then I will discuss ways in which the mother herself may be contributing to the problem without even realizing it. After presenting these potential problems, I will offer solutions that proved effective for the thousands of nursing mothers I assisted through the years.

---

[2] "Latching on," for those unfamiliar with the term, refers to when a nursing infant opens his mouth wide enough to take in not only the entire nipple far back into his mouth, but also the areola around it. He then "seals" his lips around that wide area, thus creating suction.

CHAPTER 2

Reasons Why Newborns May Have Difficulty (or Reluctance) Nursing

One of the most obvious reasons a newborn might not latch on to his mother's nipple once returned to the breast after a successful first feeding is because his mouth has had a chance to dry out, and often his mother's nipple is dry and of a substantially different texture (and shape) than what he was used to in the womb. Also, a lot more energy is now needed to obtain a trickle of fluid than when the amniotic fluid automatically rushed in without his having to suck—and that fluid now tastes different as well. If the nipple is dry, he will not suck. There will be no stimulus there. Furthermore, if his mouth is dry, his sucking reflex is not stimulated.[3]

A healthy newborn's instinctive reflexes are very strong, governing most of his activity in the first month of life. These reflexes include

---

[3]Although more will be said about bottle-feeding at the end of this booklet, I contend that one of the main reasons an artificial nipple sometimes stimulates a newborn's sucking reflex when his mother's nipple doesn't is because there is always ready moisture at its tip.

"Because most newborns lack the coordination and/or stimulation for the continuous, rhythmic sucking action that is necessary in order to successfully nurse, it takes time and patience to 'train' them in this new activity."

rooting, sucking, sneezing, gagging, coughing, and thrusting his tongue out in what is called the "extrusion" reflex. These reflexes appear cyclical as well. For instance, the newborn will nuzzle around the breast, seeking a nipple. He may turn his head back and forth in a restless motion, called rooting (which he has been practicing the last few months before birth).[4] Once he finds something to suck, he will attempt to latch on and nurse, but he almost immediately spits it out and goes back to rooting. Sometimes he may cry before beginning to suck again.

Interestingly, some modern-day mothers and nurses claim that one of the reasons newborns might be reluctant to nurse is due to the epidurals or other pain medications mothers may have received prior to delivery; they argue that these medications cause the infant to be too drowsy to nurse. Others insist that the babies are suffering a form of "withdrawal" from these drugs, resulting in restlessness and the inability to latch on and/or focus while feeding. However, I want to point out that this very behavior (restless rooting, the extrusion reflex, and a marked resistance to latching on) was vividly described by Dr. Joseph B. DeLee in his popular 1904 textbook, *Obstetrics for Nurses*, long before the advent of epidurals or modern pain medications.

Regardless, this (nonproductive) rooting activity can be very

_____

[4] Those quick, short quivering sensations many expectant mothers experience in their wombs during their last trimester is thought by some experts to be caused by the fetus rooting for his "thumb nipple."

trying for a mother who is anxious to nurse her child. She worries about hurting him if she prevents him from turning away from the nipple—especially if she is a new mother who has never held a newborn before.

Because most newborns lack the coordination and/or stimulation for the continuous, rhythmic sucking action that is necessary in order to successfully nurse, it takes time and patience to "train" them in this new activity. Some newborns catch on more quickly than others, of course, while some babies experience difficulty because the act of nursing itself is uncomfortable. Very often a newborn's tiny nose and/or forehead is tender from squeezing through the vaginal opening during delivery.

Because it takes the human body a while to register pain (especially soreness), the baby's nose isn't necessarily tender immediately after delivery. This helps explain why a newborn may nurse so readily at first but show reluctance later on: By then his nose is sore. It only makes sense that if a newborn associates pain with his breastfeeding efforts then he will resist such "feedings" and perhaps prefer a bottle instead—where nothing is pressing against him.

Depending on the size of the mother's breast and the length of her nipple, it may be that the baby can't get as close as he needs in order to latch on to the nipple without "bumping" his tender nose. Such a seemingly minor discomfort can seriously impede a newborn's attempts to nurse. Because an infant can *only* breathe through his nose the first month or so after birth, it is essential that the baby's nasal passage not be blocked in any way. Sometimes, if a newborn is strong enough, he'll push away from the nipple simply because he's having difficulty breathing; his nose is pressed too tightly up against his mother's breast. If the baby's nose is swollen from delivery, or full of excess mucus the

> "[A] newborn should nurse every 1 to 3 hours (timed from the beginning of each feeding) and not go more than 4 hours between feedings, even during the night."

first few days, his ability to breathe is inhibited, thus causing nursing difficulties as well.[5]

Sometimes a newborn may be reluctant to nurse right away because he has already "tanked up" on fluid prior to being born. Consequently, his tiny stomach is already full and he does not feel hungry. I suggest this theory because of the thousands of births I witnessed. In those cases where the mother's water broke long before delivery, or the doctor artificially ruptured the membrane at the beginning of a long labor, the infants were far more "fussy" after birth and would often drink thirstily, as though they were dehydrated. In those cases where the water broke only shortly before delivery, the babies seemed less inclined to nurse immediately. I contend that they simply weren't "hungry" yet. Also, some infants swallow a lot of air (along with mucus) upon birth, and this can make them feel "full" because their stomachs *are* full—full of air, mucus, and residual amniotic fluid.

Another reason the newborn might resist nursing is because the *feel* of his mother's nipple is very different than the types of "nipples" he sucked on in the womb, all of which supplied ample fluid without his having to actively "nurse." Considering that an infant of 5 or 6 months often has difficulty accepting an artificial (i.e., bottle) nipple if he has only been breastfed since birth, it's no wonder that a newborn might have difficulty adjusting to a

---

[5] For those mothers who choose to give birth at home, they should be aware that any infant born with a congenitally blocked nose (*choanal atresia*) requires emergency surgery so that he can breathe. Infants do not develop the capacity to breathe through their mouths until at least 4 (and sometimes up to 20) weeks old.

nipple completely unlike the objects (his own body parts) that he was sucking on in the womb. The change in shape, taste, texture, and "performance" is substantial. In short, the newborn enters this world with his nursing habits already established. If it takes adults, on average, 2 weeks to break a habit and form a new one, then it's only fair to grant a newborn that much time (or even longer!) to make the adjustment to breastfeeding.

It might be useful to mention, at this point, that a newborn should nurse every 1 to 3 hours (timed from the beginning of each feeding) and not go more than 4 hours between feedings, even during the night. This means that a mother should actually wake her sleeping newborn to feed him during the day, every few hours, so that he will sleep longer at night. Some mothers make the mistake of letting their newborn sleep during the day instead of nursing at regular intervals, and then wonder why their baby is awake all night.

If the baby begins crying due to hunger, it complicates the nursing process and frustrates both mother and infant. That is why "rooming-in" can be such a helpful process in breastfeeding. When mother and newborn are resting together in the same room, the slightest stirring from her baby will wake the mother so she can call for assistance to bring the baby to her bed—especially if she has had a C-section.[6] She can then gently and quickly move herself into a comfortable nursing position before the baby begins fussing. Although it may seem that the mother won't get as much rest this way, such rooming-in might prove beneficial if it prevents the newborn from becoming overly distressed—a situation that is often far more exhausting than is not getting enough deep sleep.

---

[6]In my experience, I saw many mothers faint their first time out of bed after delivery (both vaginal and C-section deliveries), or even within the first 24 hours. So it's best to have a nurse (or family member) bring the newborn to the mother if she has not yet successfully been up and about.

Sometimes a baby doesn't appear hungry, even if it has been several hours since his last feeding. At breast, he might root around a bit and then lose interest or else fall asleep. This behavior can be caused by the newborn's tendency to swallow air when crying, or mucus when trying to clear his air passages while lying down. In such cases, the baby might not feel hungry enough to attempt nursing; as mentioned previously, his little belly is already "full" of air and/or mucus. Consequently, he may instinctively root about, but not seriously enough to latch on to the nipple. That is why it is always beneficial to "burp" a newborn *before* placing him at breast, as well as afterwards—and between sides.[7] This will give his stomach more room for his mother's milk.

Likewise, a newborn can become fussy and fretful within hours of a successful feeding simply because he needs to have a bowel movement. Often a mother will confuse his discomfort with a desire to nurse, only to be surprised and confused when her baby persistently refuses to latch on and suckle. Because he had received a steady supply of nourishment in the womb, unpleasant sensations in his stomach are new to him; they can signal either hunger *or* the need for a bowel movement. (He doesn't know the difference; all he can do to communicate his discomfort is to cry.) I often found that a newborn would act fussy until right after an evacuation. Then he would immediately fall asleep, just like he'd been fed.

Indeed, it is helpful for a mother to know that her newborn's vigorous crying is okay (as long as it doesn't last for more than 10-15 minutes). In fact, it is both normal and even "useful." Such vigorous

---

[7]Most often a newborn will fall asleep after nursing on the first side. Since it's important to have him nurse *both* breasts at each feeding, it may be necessary to wake him up. This brief interim might serve two purposes: a quick diaper change, if needed, and burping. These activities will make him more alert for nursing on the second side and allow for him to remain asleep once he's finished.

crying helps the infant to use the muscles necessary to expedite the process of expelling the *meconium*, which may be causing constipation.

> "[N}ewborns tend to startle themselves with their own uncontrolled limbs. Sights, sounds, motion, noise: All is so very different than it was in the womb."

Another thing that might prevent the newborn from readily nursing is the surprising distraction of his own limbs. A baby within the womb is not used to flailing arms and legs. Until birth, he is safely contained within a sac, with little stimulation. (Likewise, his head has always been protected from drafts.) Consequently, newborns tend to startle themselves with their own uncontrolled limbs. Sights, sounds, motion, noise: All is so very different than it was in the womb. It takes weeks for an infant to realize that the small hand waving in front of his face or bumping against his head is actually attached to his own body. That is why the old custom of swaddling an infant makes such perfect sense. A newborn feels more secure when encased. He has already been that way for the past 9 months. So it is wise for a mother to gradually extend that feeling, alternating with freedom when he's not attempting to nurse.

Likewise, a newborn is not yet used to any sounds other than his mother's steady heartbeat, her bowel sounds, or the muffled sound of her voice when she speaks. When one stops to think about it, there is a total bombardment on the senses of a newborn. No wonder it is difficult to concentrate on the new task of rhythmic sucking in order to gain fluid! Everything is different than it was in the womb.

I realize what I'm about to say here is simply an unproven theory based on my own experience, but it seems to me that newborns are often distracted by their mothers' voices at first. Because the baby within the womb always "nursed" without effort while hearing his mother talk, it is my contention that a newborn instinctively feels as though he doesn't have to suck when he hears his mother's voice. Time and time again I witnessed a newborn lose track of the nipple or stop sucking when his mother began talking to him. It was almost as though his mother's familiar voice served as a kind of soothing distraction—even when (especially when!) she was using it to urge him to nurse.

Likewise, the sound of his mother's heartbeat soothes a newborn—which is why close cuddling is encouraged, and why the cradle position *seems* so appropriate for natural nursing. However, like I already mentioned regarding the mother's voice being a possible distraction, the reassuring sound of his mother's heartbeat—at least when first training a newborn to suckle—can be a distraction as well. It can unintentionally lull him into thinking he'll receive automatic fluid, without having to work for it. He associates both the sound of his mother's voice and the rhythmic sound of her heartbeat with a steady supply of effortless fluid. In my experience, this is why the cradle position can often lull a newborn back into sleep rather than into sucking mode.

It is very common for a newborn, when returned to his mother's nipple for a second or third nursing session, to root around, grow frustrated, and never latch on. Sometimes he will finally get the nipple in his mouth and appear to suck for a brief moment or two, only to spit it out and turn his head away. If the nipple is not far enough into his mouth, so that his lips, gums, and tongue aren't grasping part of the areola (the dark part of the nipple which contains the milk), he will not receive enough fluid to keep him stimulated to suck. (*See Figure 2: Cutaway of Infant's Mouth.*) However, a newborn has difficulty moving a "foreign object" to the back of his mouth due to a safety mechanism called the *extrusion reflex*. Consequently, it is imperative to get the mother's nipple far enough back in his mouth to bypass this reflex. After all, the nipple is merely a passageway through which the milk flows; the areola must be stimulated as well in order to prompt milk flow and adequate milk production.

That is the main problem, of course. The newborn must successfully latch on to the *areola* as well as the nipple, sucking continuously and with enough rhythm so that the milk keeps coming and he is rewarded for his efforts. When the baby roots around for a time without success, then both infant and mother grow frustrated and distressed.[8]

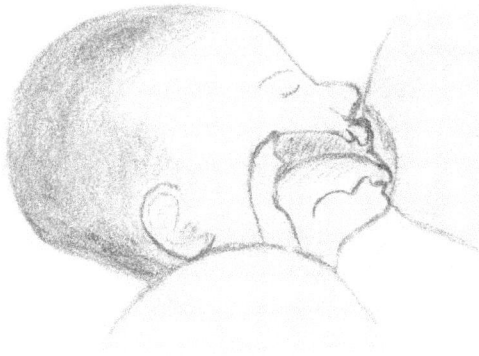

Figure 2: Cutaway of Infant's Mouth

---

[8]Newborns who are born with physical impairments that prevent successful latching on became a specialty of mine—especially after I gave birth to a daughter, early in my career, with cleft lip and palate. See Chapter 11 and my Afterward for further discussion on how to successfully nourish such infants.

CHAPTER 3

Reasons Why Mothers May Contribute to Nursing Difficulties

It is usually at this point—when the baby grows frustrated and can't seem to settle down and latch on—that the mother (unconsciously) begins contributing to the problem. As soon as she tenses up, her "letdown reflex" becomes impaired. Milk can only flow easily from a mother's breast when she is relaxed and calm. If she is frustrated, distressed, anxious, overly tired, or nervous, her body will tighten up and inhibit milk flow.

Too often I have witnessed both baby and mother become increasingly distressed when unable to nurse right away. It quickly becomes a Catch-22 situation because the milk is no longer "there" by the time the baby finally finds the nipple and begins to suck. By then the mother has become so anxious that her milk no longer easily flows, and when the newborn doesn't receive "easy" milk, he quits sucking and starts crying.

Sometimes a mother grows discouraged and frustrated due to a newborn's extrusion reflex. He will latch on to the nipple and take a few sucks but then immediately spit it out and begin rooting again or else start sucking on his own tongue. Too quickly the mother will assume he doesn't want to nurse, and she gives up on breastfeeding altogether, assuming a bottle might be easier.[9]

Usually, when this happens, the mother is simply too worried about harming the baby by holding his head gently but firmly in place until he settles into a decisive sucking pattern. I have found that mothers too often fear "persistently guiding" their infants' heads, assuming instead that a newborn will find his own way to the nipple, like he did immediately after delivery.

Sometimes it is the mother's breast and nipple size or shape that causes genuine difficulty for a baby. Very few mothers have what could be considered "perfect" nipples. Many are either flat or inverted, thus making it difficult to get enough of it into a newborn's mouth to inspire sucking. Likewise, the less protruding the nipple is, the more the baby will have to press his nose and forehead against his mother's breast in order to seize it. A newborn who is still tender in those areas will resist that effort.

Another Catch-22 for nursing mothers, in addition to the anxiety versus milk-letdown issue, is milk supply. If her baby doesn't nurse enough (or often enough), a mother's milk supply automatically dwindles. Indeed, the more frequently and completely both breasts are emptied at each feeding, the greater her milk supply. Sometimes a mother is so sore from her newborn's (unsuccessful) rooting and/ or latching on efforts that she is tempted to wait longer between feedings. It then becomes a spiral effect: The longer she waits and the less he actually drinks, the less milk there is for subsequent attempts and the more difficult it will be for him to then "find" milk.

Newborns sometimes react to the subtle changes that take place,

---

[9]As will be discussed later, in Chapter 12, a bottle is not necessarily an "easier" solution. The infant still needs to learn to latch on and actively suck in a sustained, rhythmic pattern—which means that many newborns must be taught to suck from a bottle as well. At this stage, it is not the *source* that's at issue but the *action* of sucking.

too, when a mother's milk first "comes in." (The first several days, the breasts are filled with colostrum, which has a different taste and texture than regular breast milk.) I have sometimes witnessed babies begin to resist breastfeeding after several days of successful nursing, thus causing their mothers much anxiety and even a return to the hospital to consult with a lactation specialist.

Likewise, the size and shape of a mother's nipple can sometimes change once her milk comes in, thus prompting a reaction in her newborn—especially if he is averse to change. For instance, engorgement will create a flatter-shaped nipple that is different than the one he has just learned to suckle.

Occasionally mothers will choose to give up on breastfeeding simply because it is too painful. When newborns first begin successfully sucking, they draw the nipple far back into their mouths and latch on, thus causing a lot of friction. Every time they then "lose" the nipple, that process must be undergone again, creating a great deal of tenderness and/or soreness for the mother. Sometimes the nipple becomes so painful that the mother cringes at the very thought of yet another nursing session.

This is one of the reasons why it is so very important that a mother remembers to "serve" or deliver her breast to her infant, just like she was feeding him a bottle. She needs to continue supporting her breast, holding it *still* in his mouth, so that he doesn't lose track of it.[10] If she lets go of her breast, failing to support it in his mouth, the newborn is not yet strong enough to keep enough of it in his mouth (i.e., the areola); consequently, he will only be sucking on the nipple, which does not supply milk. (Remember: The nipple

---

[10] It is important that the mother doesn't try to wiggle or move her nipple when her infant stops sucking in an attempt to stimulate him to nurse again. Doing so will cause him to lose suction.

15

"Although the cradle position is by far the most commonly pictured breastfeeding position and the one most universally associated with nursing, it is actually very difficult for a newborn to achieve."

is only a passageway.) In this situation, when he's only sucking on the nipple, it becomes a kind of non-nutritive sucking, the same as occurs with a pacifier. When this happens, a mother's nipples can become intensely sore—and her infant isn't gaining nourishment.

Sometimes a mother has difficulty with nursing due to a history of sexual abuse. These mothers are often reluctant to breastfeed or have anyone—including their babies—touch their breasts in ways that might help them grasp the nipple better. This situation can pose a very real problem, for successful breastfeeding depends on a mother being able to handle her own breasts and allow her infant access to them from various angles and positions.

Perhaps the most common and obvious cause of mothers contributing to their own breastfeeding problems, though, stems from their unrealistic expectations regarding the cradle position. Although the cradle position is by far the most commonly pictured breastfeeding position and the one most universally associated with nursing, it is actually very difficult for a newborn to achieve. It is all but impossible

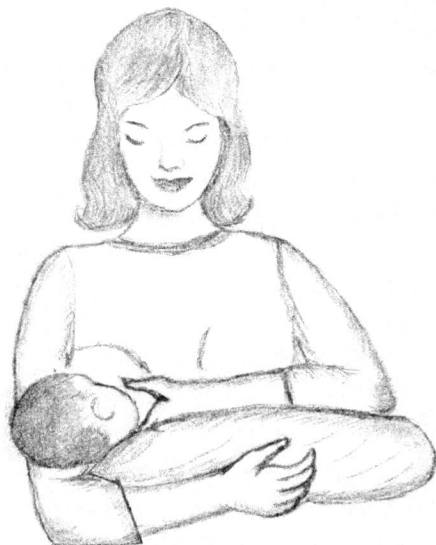

Figure 3a: Cradle Position

16

to sufficiently support a newborn's wobbly head and neck from this position, and the baby's head (often still tender from delivery) must lie against his mother's arm, creating a possibly painful distraction for him.

Likewise, a newborn's mouth may be very tiny, but it still has a distinct shape when it's open—which is always horizontal to the rest of his face. However, when the baby is lying sidewise to his mother's nipple, as happens in the cradle position, his mouth will be vertical to her nipple, and it is more difficult for a mother to one-handedly shape a vertical nipple while still cupping her breast to support it.(*See Figure 3a: Cradle Position, and Figure 3b: Vertical/Horizontal Mouth Positions.*)

Figure 3b: Vertical Mouth and Horizonal
Hand Positions

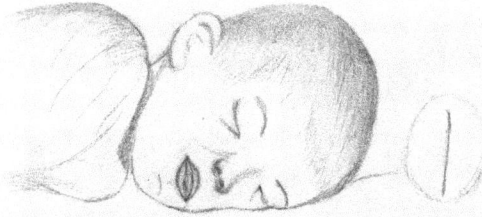

Shape of mouth when lying in cradle position

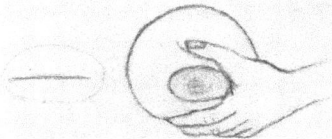

*Basic shape of nipple and
mother's left hand on breast*

17

SECTION II

Breastfeeding Solutions

The key ingredients for teaching a newborn to successfully breastfeed include staying relaxed and being persistent. It also helps to adopt other breastfeeding positions, such as the "football," "cross-cuddle," and "side-lying" positions, which I'll explain in detail later on. Likewise it is important to adjust one's expectations: Breastfeeding rarely feels "natural" to all mothers or newborns at first.

For most mothers, the act of labor and delivery are so physically draining that they need sufficient time to rest afterwards, before coping with the challenges of nursing. As mentioned earlier, the first suckle, shortly after delivery, often goes well because the baby's mouth is still moist and his sucking reflex is fully stimulated. However, it is usually during their second or third attempts to nurse that mothers and/or their newborns begin to feel frustrated. What is interesting is that these "issues" have little to do with the mother's overall experience. I have witnessed third or fourth time mothers experiencing breastfeeding difficulties; they are often dismayed that "this time" is so very different than their earlier experiences. Some newborns instinctively know how to latch on and nurse with a continuous, steady rhythm. Others must be patiently "coaxed," even over a period of days or weeks.

Consequently, the most important thing is to keep mothers relaxed and encouraged. If they are feeling anxious or worried, their letdown reflex will become severely inhibited, thus making the task even more difficult for their newborn. Listening to soothing music or drinking a favorite juice just prior to nursing tends to help calm mothers.

Very often, on his second or third attempt at nursing, the newborn will be either sleepy or fussy. In such cases, it is highly helpful for the mother to express a little of her own colostrum by hand and smear it across her nipple and areola so as to keep the area moist. Then the mother can squeeze a small amount of colostrum directly onto the baby's lips just prior to reintroducing her nipple to him. At this point, moisture is key. I often observed that the newborn would slightly close his lips to suck up that fluid, but then immediately open his mouth wide, as if to eagerly receive more. A mother should not be discouraged when her infant first closes his lips to taste the fluid she has placed there. He will soon open them again and be stimulated to start sucking. But she must be ready for this tiny window of opportunity, *for it lasts only seconds.*

If the infant has been sleeping (or crying) for a while, it is important to burp him *before* placing him at breast. Most mothers have been taught to burp a baby *after* nursing, so as to expel any bubbles that may have formed while ingesting air along with breast milk. But a newborn actually swallows a great deal of air in his first few days just while crying or lying on his back. As mentioned previously, there is also a great deal of mucous that collects in the newborn's stomach, so he can feel "full" a few hours after delivery even though he may have nursed very little. Consequently, it's wise to burp a newborn prior to nursing as well as afterwards.

❦

CHAPTER 4

Properly Burping a Newborn
& Other Helpful Tidbits

One must always keep in mind that a newborn's tiny neck is extremely flexible and weak for the first month or so after birth. This is especially true with special needs infants, such as Down's Syndrome and premature babies. Consequently, over-the-shoulder burping does not provide the kind of support these newborns need.

Because an infant's head must be supported and kept in straight alignment with his shoulders and spine, the best position for burping a newborn—and especially a premature infant—is to place him in a sitting position on one's lap, facing sideways, with one hand on his stomach, using the thumb and fingers to support his chin so it can remain steady and in alignment with his body. The other hand should support his back, gently pushing him forward while at the same time slightly patting his back to encourage burping. (*See Figure 4a: Burping Position.*) If the newborn is restless and crying,

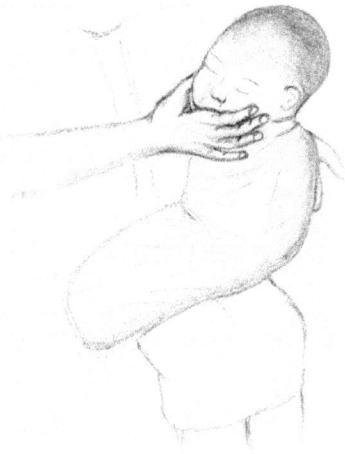

Figure 4a: Burping Position

21

however, both hands may be needed for support. In this case, one can move one's knees side-to-side and/or up-and-down in a slight rocking motion in order to gently jostle the baby. This slight movement can sometimes trigger a burp as easily as back-patting can. As long as the baby's body and head are held in straight alignment, the air should come up easily.

However, if this position *doesn't* work, then it's useful to carefully tip the baby backwards until he is lying down, in a horizontal position, making sure to keep him supported at all times. Just this change in position can encourage whatever air bubble is trapped in his stomach to rise to the front (top) of his stomach. Then gently shift him upright again, allowing the bubble to rise to the surface and all the way out.

Another tip I learned through the years that considerably helps newborns feel safe and prevents them from distracting themselves while they nurse is to swaddle them. Swaddling (i.e., wrapping a baby gently but snuggly in a soft blanket so that his arms are held close to his sides or chest) is particularly useful during initial nursing sessions, for it prevents the infant from finding his fingers or toes to suck on instead of his mother's breast.

Figure 4b: Nipple types

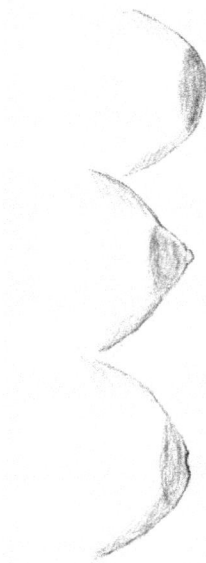

For those mothers who possess either flat or inverted nipples, it may be helpful to wear nipple shells for the last few weeks prior to delivery (*after* consulting with their doctors, of course). (*See Figure 4b: Nipple Types.*) A nipple shell is made of hard plastic and fits the contour of a woman's breast, with a hole in the center through which the nipple is "encouraged" to protrude. These shells can be worn under a woman's bra and, if positioned correctly, can help give shape to either a flat or inverted nipple. An added bonus of wearing nipple shells, I discovered, is that they can stimulate the nipple itself—which can, in turn, stimulate delivery. (That is why it is best to wait until the last few weeks of pregnancy to start wearing nipple shells, so as to not prompt early labor.)

CHAPTER 5

Breastfeeding Positions

Since the goal of those first few days of breastfeeding is to get the newborn to successfully latch on and develop a continuous, rhythmic sucking pattern, it is important to experiment with various nursing positions to find the one that most readily accommodates these two things. As mentioned earlier, one of the most common mistakes I noticed with mothers is their automatic preference for the cradle position, because this is the image they most often associate with nursing. Unfortunately, most of these depictions use older babies (2 months or more) with already established nursing patterns.

True, the cradle position does have many advantages for an infant whose nursing patterns are already well-established, for it keeps the baby's head next to the comforting sound of his mother's heart while leaving one of her hands free; it also allows for discreet nursing in public.

However, I found that this position is by far the most difficult for newborns to achieve and maintain, and I spent a lot of time coaching young mothers in a variety of other positions, including the football (or clutch), the cross-cuddle, and the side-lying. I also learned to encourage women to become comfortable supporting their own breasts by hand while their infants are nursing—at least until they learn to latch on properly and stay in a continuous, vigorous nursing pattern. Two things are accomplished by this: The infant is not as likely to tire out before getting enough milk, and the mother's nipple may not become as sore (because he will not have to suck as vigorously to keep it in his mouth).

It is imperative to remember that "tough love" parenting begins at birth. One of the main reasons so many mothers struggle with getting their newborns to properly latch on is because they are reluctant to firmly guide their babies' heads during the nursing process. It is important to keep the infant's head directed toward the breast while also supporting the nipple in his mouth. The more rooting, fussing, and crying the baby does, spitting out the nipple and "losing it," the more frustrated and sore the mother becomes, to the point that her milk flow is inhibited. This is why it is so important to find nursing positions where *both* of a mother's hands are free: one to hold her own breast so as to "deliver" it to her newborn, and the other to help guide her baby's head the first several weeks, until he is strong enough to maintain a good latch on his own.

CHAPTER 6

The Football Position

For the first few days of nursing, the football position is usually the best choice, for it enables the baby's wobbly head to be fully supported and also allows good visibility for the mother so she can see where her baby's mouth is in relation to her nipple at all times. It allows the mother to retain one hand free so she can support her breast and guide the nipple into the baby's mouth. It is also the most comfortable position if the baby was delivered cesarean, because it keeps the baby's weight off the abdominal incision. Because the baby is "sitting" in an almost upright position in this hold—and air automatically rises—the newborn may be more inclined to burp on his own, in case he hasn't been burped prior to nursing.

It is my contention that one of the reasons the football position works so well is because the newborn is sitting up and facing his mother, so he is less likely to hear his mother's heartbeat (which is a natural, soothing "lullaby" for him) and he receives less warmth this way (which helps keep him more alert). As has been mentioned earlier, the soothing sound of his mother's heart can lull a baby into thinking he doesn't have to "work" at receiving fluid. Likewise, when he is warm and cozy, he may become drowsy and lose interest in sucking. This is why, if the infant has been swaddled, it might be useful to at least uncover his head at this point; doing so will also help him become more alert.

In the football (or "clutch") hold, the baby is held similarly to how one would clutch a handbag under one's arm or a football next to one's side. The baby's head is facing the mother, upright and forward, near the breast closest to the side on which he's being held. His feet are securely tucked under his mother's arm, pointing behind her. (*See Figure 6a: Football Position.*) With the mother sitting

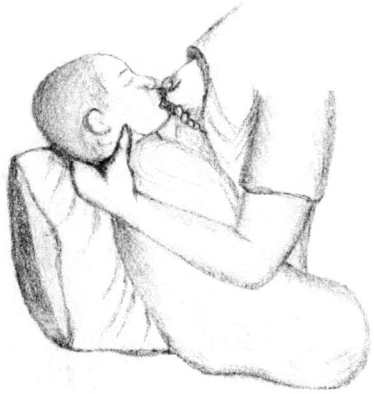

Figure 6a: Football Position

up in bed, the baby's body should be elevated by several pillows so that he can lay in a comfortable but slightly inclined position at her side and partially on her lap, facing the closest nipple. At least one pillow should be placed crosswise on her lap, very close to her, with another pillow acting as a "ramp" for the baby on the side from which she'll be nursing.

Assuming, for the sake of illustration, that the baby is on his mother's left side, then the mother's left forearm can support the newborn's upper back while her left hand clutches him to her left breast, gently supporting his shoulders, neck, and head. This frees her right hand so she can cup her breast, helping position her nipple into his mouth. (*See Figure 6b: Mother's Hands for Football Position, and Figure 6c: Close-up of Right Hand on Left Breast.*)

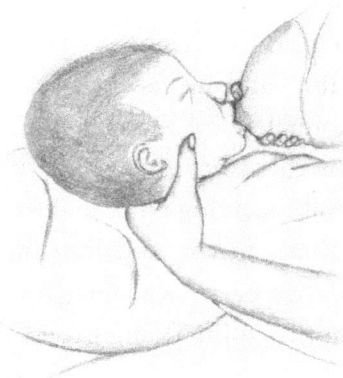

Figure 6b: Mother's Hands for Football Position

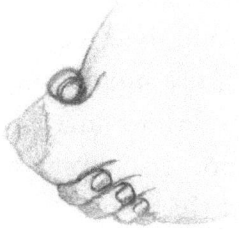

Figure 6c: Close-up of
Right Hand on Left Breast

Keeping in mind that her newborn's nose might be tender from the trauma of delivery, the mother should slightly press in the part of her breast directly under his nose with her thumb (as if he is "sniffing" her thumbnail), so that he doesn't have to bump it in order to draw enough of the nipple into his mouth. (*See Figure 6d: Top View of Football Position.*) How slightly she presses depends on how flat or inverted her nipples are, of course. With longer nipples, such pressure may not be necessary at all. In any event, the rest of her fingers need to support the breast tissue underneath her nipple, cupping her breast so as to assist her baby in getting as much of the areola in his mouth as possible—and at an angle that matches the shape of his open mouth.

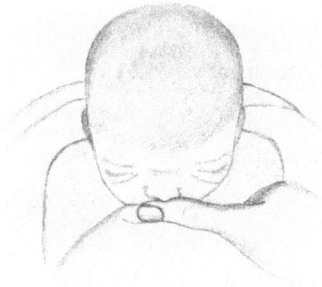

Figure 6d: Top View
of Football Position

In other words, she can create a horizontally–shaped nipple to fit his horizontally–opened mouth (as was discussed at the end of Chapter 3). This method of support will assist the newborn in keeping his mother's nipple in his mouth far more effectively than if she just trusts him to find and latch on to it by himself—like he may have done, instinctively, during his first suckle.

It is important to stress that manually supporting her breast in this manner may have to continue for *at least* two weeks—or until the baby is strong enough to find and then keep the nipple in his mouth. It has been my experience that when newborns seem to have "mastered" the art of latching on and sucking successfully, their mothers prematurely quit supporting their nipples; sooner or later, however, those infants reverted back to their old habits of losing and/or not keeping enough of the nipple in their mouths.

Some lactation specialists suggest holding the nipple like one would hold a cigarette: between the second and third fingers, with the thumb facing up. And many first-time mothers automatically do this. However, in my experience, I found that the fingers too often get in the way. Instead, I recommend using all four fingers to help cup the breast from underneath, with only the thumb pressing slightly in and down (toward the baby) from the top—what I call a modified "C" position. (*Remember: it is essential to create a slight indentation above the nipple, so that the baby's tender nose is not pressed against any flesh and has room to breathe. Of course, once the infant is no longer so tender and has mastered the art of sucking, this extra step will no longer be necessary.*)

A common mistake I saw many mothers make was to place their thumbs on the breast directly above the nipple (which is fine) but then pull backwards as the baby's mouth approached. Doing so creates a different position of the nipple, so that the baby often misses it. If the mother presses backwards with her thumb *after* the baby has already latched on, this action will usually pull the areola part of the nipple out of his mouth so that he's not getting any milk, only using the nipple as a pacifier—which, as I've mentioned before, will cause soreness. If this occurs, the mother should break the suction before pulling it out of his mouth for a new attempt. This is done by slightly pulling up his lip or by carefully placing her little finger in the corner of his mouth.

Plenty of pillows are suggested for helping to achieve the football hold, because protecting the newborn's head and/or nose from any further pressure is essential if the infant is not to associate discomfort with the nursing process. Pillows are equally important for the mother too, of course, for she needs to be as comfortable and supported as possible in order to stay relaxed. If her arms are in an awkward position, or she has to strain to keep her infant supported, she will grow tense and tired—two things that will certainly impede her letdown reflex. Remember: The newborn, once properly latched on, can nurse for up to 20 minutes at a time (approximately 10 minutes on each side), so it's important to find a position that is comfortable and sustainable for both mother and baby.

> "By supporting her own nipple in his mouth, cupping her breast so as to adapt to his mouth shape, using her other hand to gently but firmly keep him focused on her breast, and carefully indenting whatever flesh above her nipple might be pressing against his sore nose, a mother can make the task of learning to suckle a whole lot easier for her infant."

I cannot stress enough how important it is for the nursing mother to feel comfortable handling her own breast and "delivering" it to her newborn as though she were holding a bottle in his mouth during the early days of the nursing process. Many, if not most, newborns must actively *learn* to latch on and develop a rhythmic, continuous sucking pattern.[11] By supporting her own nipple in his mouth, cupping her breast so as to adapt to his mouth shape, using her other hand to gently but firmly keep him focused on her breast, and carefully indenting whatever flesh above her nipple might be pressing against his sore nose, a mother can make the task of learning to suckle a whole lot easier for

---

[11] One study I read about in *The Complete Book of Breastfeeding* claims that, out of 600 newborns, 40% had to be actively helped to suck. In my own privately-conducted, informal study, I kept track of newborns needing to be taught to suck; the numbers were similar to the official study: 35% (7 out of 20) during one period, and 42% (9 out of 21) during another. In other words, newborns had to learn the skill, and that's assuming they were physically capable of applying it once learned.

her infant. And the quicker he learns, the more contented everyone will be; he will gain nourishment faster and her nipples will be a lot less sore.

If the newborn still seems to be having difficulty latching on and successfully nursing in this football position, don't assume failure; there are other positions to try. *But first, remember the vital importance of moisture. Make sure the nipple is moist before presenting it to the newborn—regardless of the position used.*

CHAPTER 7

The Cross-Cuddle Position

Another position that works well for newborns and is similar to the football hold is the cross-cuddle position. Because this position provides even better visibility than the football hold, it can be useful for mothers who have flat or inverted nipples, extra large breasts, or newborns who are tongue-tied.[12] This position also works well if the baby is crying or cannot be consoled; more of his body is in front of (and thus closer to) the mother's center.

From the mother's perspective, the cross-cuddle position looks somewhat similar to the cradle hold—but with a significant difference. In the cradle hold, only the mother's forearm is supporting the side/top of her infant's head. In the cross-cuddle (sometimes called "transverse") position, the mother's entire arm, including her hand, is supporting the baby's back and head. It essentially involves holding the baby in a football position but placing him at her other breast, so more of his body is lying across her lap. Consequently, he

---

[12] Infants born with their tongues "tied" are far more common than many mothers expect—and can create numerous breastfeeding difficulties. About one third of the 17,000 babies I cared for after delivery had this condition. It is no longer a common practice to clip tongue-tied infants at birth. Instead, such infants are referred to specialists. The catch, though, is how best to help these infants nurse successfully *prior* to the time it takes them to see a specialist.

is lying in a more horizontal (as opposed to vertical) position. As with the football hold, a lot of pillows are required to make this position comfortable and sustainable to bring him to her nipple level so there will be no strain on his neck. (*See Figure 7a: Cross-Cuddle Position.*)

For the newborn, the cross-cuddle position is the most similar to side-lying, the position in which most newborns respond the best and which will be covered at length in the next chapter.

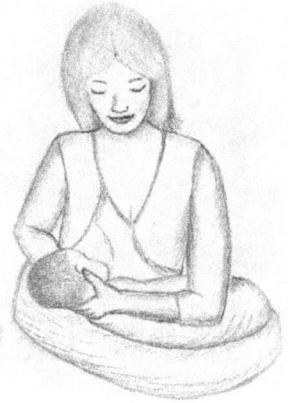

Figure 7a: Cross Cuddle

The advantage of the cross-cuddle is that the mother doesn't need assistance as much as she does for side-lying.

In the cross-cuddle position, the mother's one free hand can still cup and manipulate her breast to make her nipple into a different shape than it was in the football hold. In this position, more of the baby's body is across her lap and the mother has better visibility—particularly for a mother with large breasts and/or severely inverted nipples.

In the cross-cuddle (assuming the infant is nursing on her right breast), the mother's right elbow should be down at her side,

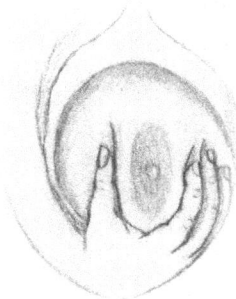

Figure 7b:

Hand Position

close to her body. Her right-hand thumb is placed on the outside of her breast with her fingers on the inside to form a vertically-shaped nipple— because her newborn's mouth will be in the vertical position lying in front of her. (*See Figure 7b: Cross-cuddle Hand Position, and Figure 7c: Cross-cuddle Top View.*) The mother's left arm and hand will be supporting his head and body. In this position, the newborn is away from the mother's warmth and heartbeat as well.

32

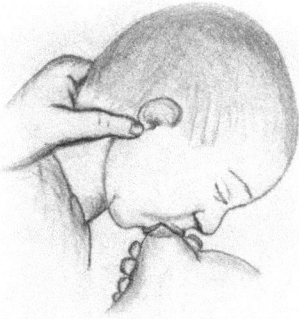

Figure 7c: Top View

The mother can support her nipple in his mouth with one hand while she firmly supports his head and body with the other. This position also applies pressure on a different part of her areola, which aids in emptying her breast completely when the various breastfeeding positions are interchanged.

As she brings her infant with her left arm up towards her nipple, she continues to support her breast and the newborn's head to keep the nipple far enough in his mouth to help him start the rhythm of nursing.

In my experience, this cross-cuddle position works extremely well for infants who have difficulty learning to latch on and/or maintain an uninterrupted period of sustained, rhythmic sucking. It is comfortable for the mother—assuming she uses lots of pillows and is well situated—and it allows her excellent visibility and control. During my many years of assisting, many infants who would not otherwise nurse found success in this position.

CHAPTER 8

The Side-Lying Position

After many attempts with the two positions mentioned so far, the mother can become discouraged if her newborn is still not readily nursing. However, she should *not* think she is a failure at this point! There is still one more position she can try: the side-lying position.

Many mothers prefer to be independent of help from a caregiver; it is only human nature to feel that way. But sometimes interdependency can be the nursing mother's most valuable option. Using my method, the side-lying position requires interdependency (at first) for the newborn who has not responded to the football or cross-cuddle positions. Before giving up on breastfeeding altogether, and choosing to rely on alternative methods of feeding her newborn, the mother should realize that this side-lying option can be especially helpful for sleepy or fussy newborns—or those who can't latch on easily. It can be very successful for teaching a newborn to accomplish the rhythm of nursing when the other positions don't work. In fact, I found that it was effective in 99% of the cases I assisted, where frustrated mothers were ready to give up on breast-feeding altogether. This position can be especially useful for mothers who are weak or need their rest. Both baby and mother are fully reclined while nursing, and although it can feel awkward at first, many mothers find this position very relaxing and enjoyable once they get used to it. This is also a very effective position for

35

night feedings.

I vividly recall a young first-time mother who was struggling to get her newborn to nurse, trying all the various positions she had learned about in breastfeeding class. After nearly an hour of unsuccessful effort, and in complete frustration, she called me for help. She was willing to let me assist her, which is essential for this position at first. Within 10 minutes, her newborn was nursing vigorously. Wonderingly, she exclaimed, "How did you learn this?" I told her it was from years of helping mothers just like her. She immediately replied, "Can you go home with me?"

The side-lying position is accomplished best with the mother lying comfortably on her side, as if she were positioning herself to sleep on whichever side she plans to nurse. If she is on her right side, she'll be nursing from her right breast. While the mother is situating herself, the "assistant" can help by holding the baby, calming him down, changing his diaper, and swaddling and/or burping him, as needed. The assistant can then carry the baby to the bed and help position him once the mother is ready.

Then, after the baby has nursed well, the mother can roll over to her other side to nurse. Again, it is best to have help in doing this, so that someone can hold the baby (and, if necessary, repeat the burping and/or changing) while she turns over and adjusts her body into a comfortable position on her left side. If a mother has not had a C-section, it should be easy to find a relaxing, side-lying position. If she *has* had a C-section, turning far enough may be uncomfortable, so it's helpful to place a firm pillow or folded blanket next to her in order to raise the infant to the level of her nipple.

Assuming the mother is lying on her right side to begin with, she will need at least one or two pillows under her head for comfort and visibility. She should turn far enough to be comfortable, allowing her right breast to rest in a natural position on the bed, straight out in front of her. The bed is the best support for the nipple in this position. If the nipple can remain steady, her infant can keep it in his

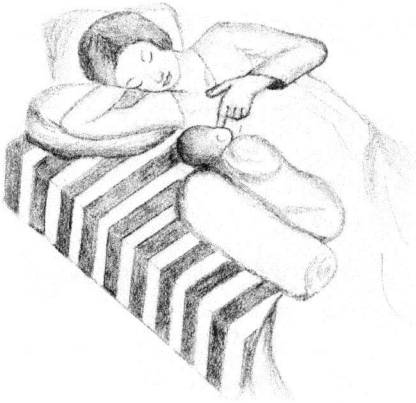

Figure 8a: Side-Lying

mouth better and nurse more easily because his head, neck, and shoulders are in straight alignment; he will be lying on his side with his mouth even with her nipple. (*See Figure 8a: Side-Lying Position.*)

The mother's right arm should be placed high enough under her head so that her infant will have nothing touching the top of his (possibly tender) head while nursing. The bed can provide firm support for the side of his head, providing less motion so that he's not distracted from finding his sucking rhythm. The assistant should reassure the mother that her newborn will not be allowed to roll away while he is placed on his side, since the assistant will be present to support and guide his head.

Experience has shown that, in this position (still assuming she's on her right side), it works best for the mother to place her left index finger on her breast (as if she were pointing) just slightly above the areola. Her index finger will be placed where the newborn's nose is positioned, making a slight dimple on her breast in front of his nose. (*See Figure 8b: Side-Lying Top View.*)

If she has flat or inverted nipples, she may have to press a little more firmly to make the nipple extrude to more of a point. Sometimes the areola is very large, so the mother may have to place her finger on it. The exact

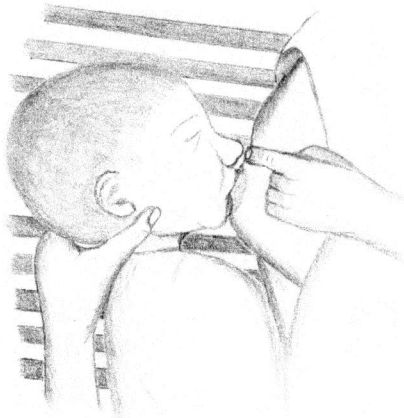

Figure 8b: Side-Lying Top View

37

placement of her finger depends entirely on how large her areola is. She should stay in that same position as the assistant gently guides the newborn to her nipple. Her index finger should go straight in and down, depending on where her newborn's nose will be after he grasps the nipple. It should remain there as he latches on. (Moving her finger out of the way of her newborn's nose will change the position of the nipple, often pulling it out of his mouth. This is especially likely to happen if he has not had time to start his rhythm of sucking.) (*See Figure 8c: Pointing Index Finger.*)

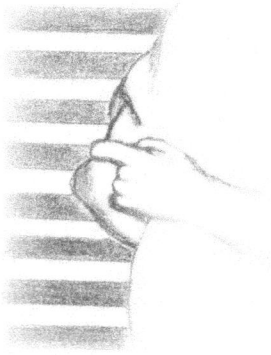

Figure 8c:
Mother's Pointing
Index Finger (Top View)

If done properly, the mother's index fingernail should be just under the newborn's nose, as if he were sniffing it, thus allowing him more room to breathe while so close to her breast. She should keep her finger in that same place the entire time he is nursing on that side. He will be able to breathe around her fingernail far easier than he can if pushed up close to her breast tissue. Remember: A newborn breathes *only* through his nose for the first month or so after birth; he is not yet able to breathe through his mouth. Hence, it is imperative to keep his nasal passages cleared and his tender and/ or swollen nose free from the potentially suffocating effect of being squished up too closely to his mother's breast.

When the mother's thumb is on top and her fingers underneath her breast, as is illustrated in most breast-feeding books, the position of her hand makes it difficult for the newborn to attach to the breast while they are both in the side-lying position. (The nipple will be horizontal to his vertical mouth.) It also makes visibility difficult for the mother: She can't clearly see what her infant is doing.

With the mother's permission, the assistant can create the same

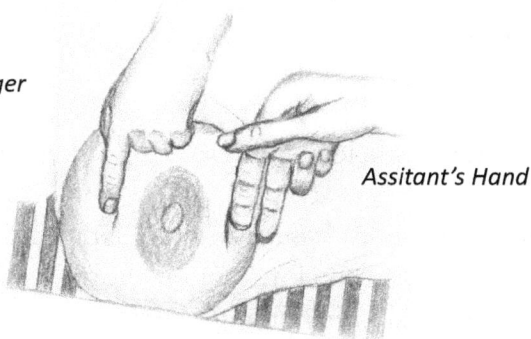

Mother's Finger

Assitant's Hand

Figure 8d:

Assisted Finger Placement

effect as the traditional thumb-on-top-fingers-underneath hand placement. This is done at the same time the mother is placing her index finger in and down toward the top of her (moist!) nipple. (Remember: Moisture is key! Dribbling a little fluid on the nipple will create necessary moisture if there is not enough manually expressed colostrum.) (*See Figure 8d: Assisted Finger Placement.*)

The assistant simultaneously supports the breast from the other side (with her right hand), helping to bring the nipple to a point. The goal is to bring the nipple straight out to the newborn, providing both room and visibility for the nipple to be placed directly into his mouth. (In this right-side lying position, the assistant's left hand will be supporting the infant's head while guiding him to the nipple.)

With the mother's index finger placed in front of the newborn's nose, and her not moving it as he grasps the nipple, the newborn can get more of the nipple into his mouth. If the nipple goes in deep enough, with most of the areola covered by his lips, the milk ducts will be emptied with the newborn's sucking—and enough fluid will be there to prompt his sucking reflex.

This is where patience on the mother's part is important. She may have to wait a minute or two for him to establish a steady nursing rhythm—which may seem like an eternity at the time—but it is worth it. The placement of her finger just under his nose prevents the newborn from letting go of the nipple, which in turn allows him the time he needs to achieve the rhythm of sucking. By staying on the nipple longer, his sucking reflexes have more time to kick in.

After the newborn has successfully latched on, and after a few minutes of successful sucking action, he will usually stop to rest. The mother should keep her finger in the same place and not move it, for this will break any suction he might have established. (The assistant's right hand should continue to support the other side of the nipple.) When the index finger remains just under his nose, even *after* he grasps the nipple and starts sucking, he will be able to keep the nipple in his mouth when he stops to rest or breathe.

Once the newborn has maintained a good sucking rhythm for a few minutes, the assistant can then carefully position his torso and hips so that his body is more in alignment with his shoulders and neck. He also won't be able to turn away as easily once he's more on his side, facing his mother. Instead of the mother bringing her arm around and possibly pressing against his tender head, it is better to tuck a folded receiving blanket under his torso and hips to keep him from rolling away when the assistant then leaves (making sure the bedrail is firmly up, if mother and child are still at the hospital).

If the infant *does* let go, the mother should remain still, with her finger in place; the newborn will then root a little bit but hopefully latch right on again. If not, she should feel free to call again for help. This is why it is important to make sure her call light is within reach, or for her assistant to return frequently to check their progress. It is best if the mother holds still and lets her newborn do the moving—up to a point, of course. Doing so will help the infant stay calm and not lose track of the nipple. If the mother moves at the same time the baby moves, they will miss each other's "target"—her nipple. I had to remind mothers of this fact time and time again. It is best for the mother to remain still while the baby finds his way back to her nipple. If he still has the nipple in his mouth but is not sucking, the assistant can stimulate him to begin nursing again by simply rubbing his back or lightly tickling his feet. Also, a little dribble of moisture into the corner of his mouth can prompt his sucking to start again.

Once a newborn's nursing habits are successfully established and he is getting maximum milk flow, this index finger method does not have to be continued. The other position of the mother's hand on her nipple will work because, by then, his head and nose are less tender.

As mentioned earlier, it takes more initial effort—and the help of an assistant—to begin nursing in the side-lying position, but I found that it was the surest way to achieve a successful latching on and sustained rhythmic nursing pattern for those infants for whom other breastfeeding positions were not successful. For one thing, being able to lie in a side position can be very restful and relaxing to an exhausted, recently-delivered mother. Having an assistant help manage the infant's position can assist her enormously so that she can focus on relaxing. Likewise, it has been established that infants are much more alert when lying on their sides. (Again, this perhaps has to do with the newborn not being able to hear—and then be lulled asleep by—his mother's heartbeat and/or his not receiving direct warmth from his mother.) Furthermore, this is the only breast-feeding position in which there is nothing touching the infant except for the slight pressure from the bed—which provides a steady support. He can lie perfectly still and have the breast delivered to him. This win-win combination of a relaxed mother and a comfortable but alert baby makes for optimal nursing conditions.

CHAPTER 9

Breast Care

Often, when a mother's milk first comes in, her breasts engorge to the point that her nipple size and shape changes substantially, and the baby, if he is averse to change, will fuss. Even though the flow rate will be much higher than it was with colostrum, so that the baby "gets more" for his effort, the nipple can become flatter, thus making it more difficult for him to latch on.

In such cases, it is wise for the mother to express some milk prior to nursing so that her nipple is softer and more elongated and the baby can get more of it into his tiny mouth. Because the letdown reflex can take up to 7 minutes or more, sometimes pumping the breast for (only!) a few minutes immediately before nursing helps. This will alleviate pressure and soften the nipple; it can also stimulate flow, so that when the baby latches on there is a ready supply of milk. Placing a warm washcloth on the breast can also stimulate milk flow, bringing the milk closer to the surface.

Mothers should always begin nursing their newborns on whichever breast they last suckled. Here is the reason: A newborn usually nurses more vigorously on the first side he's given, and for longer. That first side consequently empties more completely than the second because the baby is either too sleepy or too full by then to finish. Hence, it's important to alternate the breasts that are first introduced; otherwise, one breast will begin producing more milk than the other.

It is also essential to nurse (and/or breast-pump) equally on both sides with each feeding in order to stimulate the hormone that tells the mother's body to produce more milk. If a mother is not producing enough milk, it might be necessary to revisit the doctor to make sure that all the placenta was removed during the afterbirth, for even one small piece of placenta left in the uterus tells the body that the baby is not yet born and thus hinders the action of the hormone that stimulates milk production.

Once the baby is nursing readily and successfully, it is wise for a mother to alternate the various breastfeeding positions as well. Such frequent changes can help prevent sore nipples because the pressure of the infant's sucking changes to different parts of her nipple, depending on his position. Likewise, different parts of her milk ducts will receive stimulation and pressure, thus encouraging each of them to empty thoroughly.

It is common for mothers to get mastitis, which is caused from bacteria entering into any open and/or bleeding cracks in the nipple area. So keeping the nipple soft and air-dried is of utmost importance. (Warmth and moisture feed bacteria.) If the cracks persist, one can administer an edible cream, available over the counter at most drug stores. Keep in mind, of course, that some infants might resist the taste of such creams—but preventing cracks is imperative.

When All Else Fails

If, after all these breast-feeding positions are attempted, the newborn is still not gaining weight as he should, he will need supplemental nourishment. This raises the complicated and sometimes controversial issue of how to gain that nourishment. However, it is deeply important to stress at this point that a mother should NEVER feel like a failure because she's had to resort to alternative methods of feeding! Sometimes other options must be considered in order to assure adequate nutrition, and doing so in no way reflects on a mother's skills or abilities.

CHAPTER 10

Nipple Confusion
Versus Fluid Confusion

Through my many years of nursing, I have seen various trends come and go regarding infant care and nursing advice. For years, we delivery and neonatal nurses were allowed to give bottles to newborns in the nursery while their exhausted mothers rested and/or caught up on their sleep. While using my methods, I never once saw a baby refuse the breast after receiving a bottle-feeding at night while his mother slept. (Whereas I did observe that babies who had not received a bottle in the nursery often had difficulty learning to breastfeed.) Indeed, the "practice" of sucking on even an artificial nipple seemed to *enhance* the baby's ability to latch on and rhythmically suck his mother's breast. Likewise, a baby who received supplemental nutrition at night, prior to being placed back at his mother's breast for his next attempt at natural feeding, was usually stronger, more alert, and thus more amenable to nursing. Both mother and baby were more satisfied.[13]

---

[13] Interestingly, we nurses observed that "bottle babies" (those infants who—for whatever reason—weren't able to breastfeed) frequently had to be taught to suck on an artificial nipple during the first 24 hours after birth. To me, such behavior suggests that it isn't the nipple itself that's the problem so much as learning how to latch on and suck in such a way as to gain fluid. Some infants just learn more quickly than others, regardless of the "delivery system" (i.e., nipple).

"Indeed, the 'practice' of sucking on even an artificial nipple seemed to *enhance* the baby's ability to latch on and rhythmically suck his mother's breast."

By the late 1950s, though, when so many mothers had begun to rely on the convenience of bottle-feeding, there was a trend to return to "nature's way." Rates for breastfeeding had dropped to the all-time low of 20%, and La Leche League (LLL) was formed, with its inspiring determination to encourage mothers to only breastfeed their newborns. Consequently, it became increasingly unpopular to provide bottles in hospital nurseries—for fear of something lactation professionals called "nipple confusion." By the mid-1980s, it became standard hospital protocol to discourage giving all newborns the bottle.[14]

Although I have yet to see any studies proving there actually is such a thing as nipple confusion, the trend for the past 25 years or so has been to avoid introducing an artificial nipple to a newborn while he's still learning to breastfeed for fear he might reject his mother's breast in favor of the bottle. This theory has become so widespread that it now poses as fact, and both bottles and pacifiers were practically banned from most hospital nurseries years ago. While I was still assisting deliveries in the mid-2000s, a nurse could actually get "written up" for supplying a bottle to calm a fretful infant when the mother was asleep or otherwise unavailable for nursing.

What seems so ironic about this policy is that experience simply doesn't back it up. For instance, many Latina mothers used to insist (back when they were allowed to do so) on giving a bottle immediately after breastfeeding if their babies were still fussing, for they assumed their infants hadn't received enough. (I

---

[14] And this trend continues! At present, there is even talk in Congress about giving breastfeeding mothers a "tax rebate."

always encouraged them to give the bottle immediately so that it wouldn't interfere with their newborns' appetites come next feeding time.) Consequently, these women bottle-fed their newborns immediately after nursing and yet had no difficulty

> "In my opinion, babies have not changed much over the centuries—only the 'experts' have."

in transitioning them back to the breast. Where is the nipple-confusion there?

However, this rampant fear of bottle-feeding has gradually morphed into protocols at some hospitals that are geared more for nurses' standards-of-practice than for teaching mothers specific methods that will help them start breast-feeding their newborns. Underlying these new "policies" is a strict taboo against using any artificial nipple or pacifier. When I recently asked a lactation specialist why this is, she said, "We don't know which newborn might develop confusion; therefore, no newborn should experience an artificial nipple."

In my opinion, babies have not changed much over the centuries—only the "experts" have. As mentioned previously, an obstetrics textbook written by Dr. DeLee in 1904 described the same breast-feeding problems I observed a century later. Indeed, archeologists have discovered ancient "baby bottles" dating back to 500 B.C. If nursing was so "natural" back then—prior to hospitals, modern medicine, and professional lactation consultants—why the need for bottles?

Likewise, there is a long history of wet nurses.[15] If nipple confusion truly exists, then wouldn't infants experience problems switching back and forth between human nipples as well? (The

---

[15] And even goats! Several history books of breast-feeding I've consulted contain depictions of infants directly nursing from goats.

size, shape, and texture of human nipples vary widely.) A story I read recently on the internet about breastfeeding problems told of a woman who served as a modern day "wet nurse" to help a 4-day-old who was having trouble breastfeeding with his mother. This woman, who was lactating at the time, had no trouble getting the infant to nurse from her own breasts; on the very first attempt, he got the hang of it and was easily transferred back to his grateful mother, who experienced no further difficulties.

I sometimes feel like the lone voice in a crowd by suggesting that it is not "nipple confusion" at all as much as it is "fluid confusion"—if there even *is* any confusion. The adjustment a newborn must make between passively receiving fluid *around* one of his "thumbs" in the womb (or via a feeding tube after birth) and learning to actively suck nourishment *through* a nipple (which requires stimulation) is significant. Those infants who receive passive nourishment—such as spoon, cup, or finger/tube feeding— are not developing the muscle tone, suction, coordination, and calming rhythmic patterning of actively breastfeeding babies. Time and time again I've seen newborns who, because they were not allowed a bottle for fear of "nipple confusion," were forced to use these passive alternative methods their first few days of life.

This current practice concerns me for a number of reasons, not least of which is that most of these lactation specialists and breastfeeding "professionals" are not old enough to remember the days when bottles were allowed in the nursery and were actually used to assist in helping newborns learn to nurse. These present-day nurses grew up and received their training under the assumption that bottles are "bad" and nipple confusion is real. Many of them now go to extreme measures to make sure no artificial nipple of any kind is introduced to a newborn, regardless of common sense. They contend that the newborn uses different muscles for the bottle compared to what he needs for accessing his mother's nipple. But my question is: Didn't he use different muscles on his thumbs and fingers before birth?

Consequently, this current "anti-bottle" trend poses a real challenge for those unfortunate newborns who simply cannot breastfeed due to a variety of physical limitations.

CHAPTER 11

Special Needs Infants

In addition to the problems I've already cited in earlier chapters as to why newborns might have difficulty nursing, some infants just aren't physically capable of receiving adequate nourishment from a mother's breast. Some babies arrive prematurely and aren't yet strong enough to nurse on their own. Others are born with deformities, such as cleft lip and/or palate, precluding the ability to create a strong enough suction to supply adequate nourishment. Some infants have low blood sugar at birth and are too weak to sustain a sucking pattern. Many Down's Syndrome infants lack the muscle tone needed to effectively nurse. These "special needs" newborns require a different approach to feeding, and most of the measures used in hospitals today replicate the kind of passive fluid intake they received in the womb, when the amniotic fluid flowed into their open mouths whilst they "sucked" on their thumbs, fingers, or other body parts.

These types of passive feeding methods—such as tube-feeding, "finger"-feeding, and the cup and spoon method—rely on the newborn simply swallowing fluid placed inside his mouth that then trickles in *around* the finger. Instead of the milk coming through a portal that the newborn must actively "suck on," the milk seeps in around the object. In this way, the infant does not need to latch on or create suction. For some infants, this is the only way they might be able to gain nourishment at first, until they are strong enough to actively suck, thus replicating how they received fluid in the womb. But at some point, once (and if) they are able, these infants will still have to learn to latch on and actively suck in a rhythmic, sustained manner—be it at their mothers' breasts or with bottles (i.e., natural or artificial nipples).

Having given birth to a daughter with severe cleft lip and palate when I was only 23 and just beginning my career as a neonatal nurse, I experienced firsthand the anxiety of a mother desperate to nourish her newborn but unable to do so. Suddenly, my experience in the delivery room and in assisting other mothers with nursing problems no longer helped. The only way we could get milk into the gaping "hole" that was my poor baby's mouth those first two terrifying weeks was with a small medicine dropper that held a teaspoon of formula. We had to be careful she didn't choke, and her extrusion reflex often caused her to spit the formula right back out. She was eventually fitted with a removable artificial palate that (inadvertently) enabled her to create suction so she could "nurse" from a Brecht Feeder, a customized device for special needs infants. This Brecht Feeder has since been replaced by the Haberman Feeder, which has been quite successful for a number of years—albeit expensive.

The desperation I felt during those early days, combined with my subsequent years of assisting all kinds of mothers to nurse all kinds of newborns, resulted in the creation of this booklet—as well as the invention of a revolutionary new feeding device to assist similarly distraught parents of special needs infants. It is an affordable alternative to the Haberman Feeder and helps even cleft lip and palate babies achieve suction so they can actively nurse rather than rely on passive feeding methods.

After all, true "nursing" requires the ability to simultaneously coordinate breathing, sucking, and swallowing—no small feat. And, as I've mentioned previously, this method of obtaining nourishment is far different from the passive feeding an infant experiences in the safety of the womb.

Back in the days when bottle-feeding newborns was still popular, I learned firsthand that at least half of the newborns we had to feed in the nursery resisted the bottle nipple at first. It didn't seem to matter if it was their mothers' natural nipples or the artificial nipples we were using in the nursery; many of these newborns simply resisted having to actively suck in order to gain fluid. We literally had to teach them. I observed, again and again, that once the newborn associated latching on and rhythmic sucking with obtaining fluid—whether with a bottle or at his mother's breast—he would continue to do fine with either.

> "It didn't seem to matter if it was their mothers' natural nipples or the artificial nipples we were using in the nursery; many of these newborns simply resisted having to actively suck in order to gain fluid."

It wasn't until after the infant had breastfed successfully for some weeks (or months) and was first transitioned to the bottle that resistance occurred—especially when the mother had to return to work or had to stop nursing due to illness or other circumstances. But even these babies quickly got the hang of it within a short amount of time and were successfully nourished by either means.

No, it is the special needs infants—those who simply *can't* create suction or who aren't strong enough to actively nurse—that require passive feedings at first. To force such measures on infants who are capable of learning to latch on and rhythmically "suck" simply because of a fear of the *possibility* of nipple confusion seems ludicrous to me.

⁕

CHAPTER 12

How Artificial Nipples Can Help

As I've already mentioned, most lactation specialists today are reluctant to provide nourishment even to a weak newborn via a bottle for fear he will then prefer it over his mother's nipple—for it is often believed that bottle feeding is "easier" for an infant, even though the mechanics of sucking are the same.[16]

To me, such thinking just seems wrong-headed—and even dangerous. As a highly regarded pediatrician once told us at a nurses' conference in the early 1990s, "If a newborn has not nursed successfully within 24 hours after birth, the mother should pump her milk out and give it to the infant in a bottle." This doctor was widely known at that time as the "guru of breastfeeding." And yet, even she advised common sense when it came to caring for a struggling newborn. The longer the infant goes without feeding, the weaker he becomes, and the harder it then is to learn to suckle.

For instance, those babies who are born with low blood sugar, thus causing them to be lethargic and weak, often have difficulty breastfeeding at first; they are just too tired to make the effort.

---

[16] If a newborn seems to prefer the bottle nipple, it may be that the bottle does not press against his tender nose. Or perhaps he simply feels more "at home" with a bottle nipple because it is shaped more like his in-womb "thumb nipple." As I mentioned in footnote 3, on p. 3, I suspect some infants are more stimulated by a bottle simply because of the ready moisture at its tip.

57

Getting a little colostrum into them right away will help regulate the imbalance and give them energy so they can suckle. Because a bottle nipple provides more rapid flow than a mother's breast and is sometimes easier for an infant to manage, it makes sense to provide nourishment for the baby in this manner, quickly, so that he can become strong enough to nurse. The mother can hand-express or pump some of her colostrum that is then delivered to the newborn via a soft, artificial nipple. By having to "suck" this nipple in order to receive fluid, the baby will be better prepared for breastfeeding. This step could be compared to using "training wheels" when learning to ride a bike. For some children, such an intervening step is necessary. Passive methods for gaining nourishment are not nearly as convenient or effective—nor do they teach the newborn to *actively suck*. Likewise, there is always a danger of choking when using passive feeding methods; a newborn can't readily swallow fluid that is being dribbled (at someone else's will) into their open mouths.

I was delighted to learn, when talking to a farmer friend one day, that her method of getting baby lambs to nurse was very similar to some of the "tricks" I employed when assisting newborns to latch on. My friend mentioned that she would often have to help guide a wobbly-legged newborn lamb to the nipple and squirt a little milk onto its muzzle to "give it the scent." Sometimes the lamb would resist, choosing to suck instead on a tag of wool nearby its mother's teat. She would have to gently force the lamb's focus onto the nipple, sometimes even "stuffing it" into its little mouth. She assured me that baby lambs could be just as stubborn and seemingly "clueless" about nursing as the human newborns I'd attended.

She admitted that she often guided a lamb's mouth by wetting her little finger with colostrum and then getting the lamb to "follow it" to the nipple. She would sometimes even get the lamb to suck on her finger briefly as she moved her finger closer and closer to the mother's nipple—until the "bait-n'-switch" was successfully completed.

Because she often had a bottle on hand for feeding older lambs that needed extra nourishment, she quickly learned that she could simply use the wet bottle nipple (making sure it was warm and slathered with its mother's fresh colostrum) as a kind of "bait." She would entice the lamb to suck by rubbing the moist bottle nipple across its lips; as soon as the lamb began to work its mouth around the nipple and begin sucking, she would move the bottle nipple towards the mother's nipple, making a quick "trade" when the two nipples were side by side.

This procedure is very similar to what we night nurses sometimes did with mothers who needed help breastfeeding their newborns. For infants who were fussy and couldn't seem to latch on, we could actually quiet them down and get them started nursing by using a bottle. As soon as the infant was calmly latched on and beginning to suck, we would simply transfer him to his mother's nipple. The newborn would then continue sucking vigorously. It was soothing for both baby and mother, and I never once saw an instance of "nipple confusion."

Indeed, as I mentioned earlier, an infant who has only breastfed for the first few months of life must learn to adjust to a bottle when (or if) it is finally introduced to him. It depends, of course, on his openness to change, but some infants experience difficulty in adapting to a bottle and must seemingly be "taught" to nurse all over again. In such cases, I found

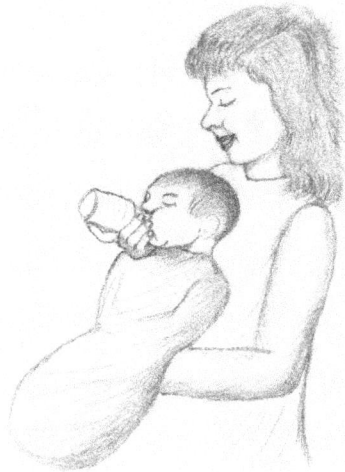

Figure 12:
Bottle-feeding Facing Out

that it helps to position the infant facing "outward" when doing so. (*See Figure 12: Bottle-feeding Facing Out.*) Again, as in breaking old habits from the womb, it is important to disrupt the infant's old associations. By having the infant facing outwards, rather than toward the breast, the baby is distracted and will be less likely to expect his nourishment to be received in the same way. I have found that he is likewise more amenable to a new experience if he's not in his usual nursing position.

The fuss over nipple confusion seems to have spread to pacifiers, too. They are currently discouraged until the infant has successfully learned to breastfeed and is at least 2 to 4 weeks old. Some professionals also suggest that infants sucking on pacifiers will be less inclined to nurse and thus won't stimulate their mothers' milk supply as much. Again, I can say from experience that a mother's milk will "come in" regardless of whether her infant is breastfeeding or not, and a baby will experience hunger and the need to nurse whether or not he's finding nonnutritive enjoyment from sucking a pacifier. True, the supply might be less if the infant is not nursing as much, but there is no way that a pacifier alone will cause a baby not to nurse. What's important is how and when the mother chooses to use it.

The oddest part of this argument against pacifiers, from my point of view, is the assumption that they will "confuse" the newborn. It has already been established that a baby has been using various "pacifiers" in the womb, before birth. He associates the intake of fluid with this nonnutritive sucking action, and the practice soothes him. Besides, a newborn will readily find something to suck on, regardless of whether or not he has successfully learned to latch on to his mother's nipple and attain milk. He usually will find a thumb or finger, so how is an artificial pacifier any different? Likewise, many a mother will automatically slip her little finger into her newborn's mouth to help calm him—a pacifying action that the "specialists" don't yet forbid. Studies have even shown that the use of pacifiers can reduce the risk of SIDS when putting a baby to sleep during naps or at bedtime, and pacifiers help calm fretful infants.

I learned in nurses' training that "the act of sucking is essential for an infant in order to feel secure." These words came to haunt me when my own cleft lip and palate daughter was born a few years later. She couldn't suck! Consequently I spent endless hours holding and rocking her every day in an effort to make sure she felt safe. It was bad enough that we couldn't seem to get enough nourishment into her via passive feeding methods, but it terrified me to think that she might feel insecure as a newborn because she wasn't able to experience the comfort of "sucking."

In short, pacifiers are extremely useful, and it seems downright silly to deprive a newborn of one just because he "might" develop nipple confusion. They help the infant calm down, and the sucking action they induce creates perastolic waves in the gastro-intestinal system to aid in the passing of gas or stools. We often would use pacifiers on newborns in the hospital nurseries before such practice was "outlawed." Again, I feel like I'm the lone voice in the crowd who is willing to talk about the "good old days" when we were able to keep newborns pacified and nourished in the nursery while their mothers caught up on much-needed rest. In my experience, a bottle and/or pacifier actually *assisted* the infant in learning to breastfeed and made for a more comfortable experience for all involved.

"In short, pacifiers are extremely useful, and it seems downright silly to deprive a newborn of one just because he 'might' develop nipple confusion."

Conclusion

Yes, I definitely agree that mother's milk is best and that breastfeeding is by far the healthiest, most "natural" way to nourish newborns and help establish that wonderful mother-child bond. But I wrote this little booklet because of (and for!) the extraordinary number of mothers who find that those initial days of breastfeeding aren't nearly as easy as they expected them to be. I'm also deeply sensitive to the plight of mothers who somehow feel like "failures" as mothers because they can't breastfeed—either because their infants are unable to do so or because they themselves have problems that preclude nursing.

As I've made clear in this booklet, the best solutions were simply trying other breastfeeding positions and letting go of those unrealistic expectations regarding the cradle position. The only "failures" I ever encountered in helping a newborn to breastfeed was when the mother simply didn't have the will to nurse, or gave up prematurely. I discovered early on that "tough love"—successful parenting—starts at the beginning, with nursing. Like I always told my patients: "The labor doesn't end with delivery; your job has only just begun!"

But our efforts were always worth it. One day recently I ran into a mother I had once helped to breastfeed. She was with her preteen daughter—the very child that needed my assistance early one morning a few days after she'd gone home from the hospital. After thanking me, again, for all my assistance those many years ago, the mother turned to her daughter and exclaimed: "If it wasn't for this lady, you would've starved to death!"

Afterward

As I've mentioned earlier in this booklet, I have actually designed and patented a radically new feeding device that replicates a mother's real nipple and can be used on either special needs infants, as a way of getting fluid into them the "natural" way, or normal newborns, as a pacifier. I call it the YUM Feeder (Your Utter Magic), and it will soon be available for sale online.

The inspiration for my invention came one night while I was at work. My coworker and I were discussing the problems of breastfeeding mothers, and their fear of nipple confusion. We both agreed that a newborn needed a nipple that would feel just like a mother's so there would no longer be any possibility of "confusion." As I've mentioned earlier, we delivery and neo-natal nurses know from experience that providing an occasional bottle or pacifier to newborns can actually *help* them learn to suck and, if done properly, serve as an aid to the breastfeeding process. It distressed many of us nurses to see bottles so vehemently banned from hospitals due to this fear of nipple confusion.

If only we could get an artificial nipple to be more like a mother's breast!

If we could do so, many of these struggling newborns could learn to suck using an example most like their mothers'. After all, "wet nurses" were now out of fashion (at least in the States), and passive methods of feeding, such as the cup and spoon, do not help newborns learn the art of sucking the "natural" way.

While I was drawing up possible nipple designs and researching how to obtain a patent, my manager called me at home. She asked whether I knew of a product that a new baby with a cleft lip and palate could use to help satisfy its sucking needs. I told her there really were none for that purpose available. The feeders I had used with my daughter (and had seen during the years since she had grown) had the usual nipple shape. At that point my original design ideas changed.

My thoughts went back to my daughter's difficult and long first feedings with a small medicine dropper during her first two weeks of life. Because of her cleft lip and palate, the opening in her mouth and gums was wide enough to slip my index finger through. As a nurse, I had already experienced trying to feed newborns with that defect, but this was different: It was my own daughter, and her opening was wider than any I had ever seen. The struggle experienced in feeding her was far different from those I had with the babies on my job.

The small hospital where I delivered her had only been able to provide a medicine dropper. But her gag reflex was such that she would automatically spit out anything we tried to dribble into her mouth—and/or choke. I eventually gained access to a Breck Feeder—which acts more like a syringe—and we were semi-successful in getting nourishment into her that way, but only after a surgeon's help.

She needed surgery, of course, but the doctor's first comment to us two weeks after she was born disheartened me: "We think we can fix her." I had been hoping to hear, "We *know* we can fix her." The doctor said he wanted to try a new experiment for the purpose of drawing her gums together so that, after the surgery, there would be less scarring. I remember him saying, "She is a pretty girl, and should get all the dividends."

This "experiment" (which they still use to this day) involved making a hard plastic plate—somewhat like a denture plate but with no teeth in it—that would fit over her gums and "cover" the hole in her palate. It was intended to simply draw her gums together to prepare for surgery—which she finally received at 22 weeks old.

However, shortly after we got her home with this new device, I heard small smacking sounds while she slept. The plate inadvertently allowed her to achieve suction, and her feedings consequently became much easier because she could use her own rhythm of sucking. What serendipity! The doctor had designed it for one purpose, but it also accomplished another.

My daughter ended up requiring 16 more surgeries over the next 23 years in order to have a normal mouth and smile, and I'm proud of what a strong, beautiful, self-confident woman she has become. But I couldn't help thinking of all the cleft lip and palate babies born in countries where surgery is not readily available—or affordable. As it was, we needed two incomes and lots of loans in order to pay for all those surgeries. What happens to infants without that option? How do they get nourished?

Many don't, of course. The infant mortality rate in developing nations is staggering—and special needs infants are the first to die. There is simply no way to feed them.

Consequently, when trying to design a natural nipple that replicated a mother's breast so as to minimize any fear of nipple confusion, I couldn't help but recall my daughter's experience with that experimental "plate," and how it unexpectedly fostered her ability to gain suction—the very thing necessary to latch on and nurse rhythmically. I thus designed and patented a flexible, leak-proof nipple that provides even cleft lip and/or palate babies with enough "coverage" to enable suction. Shortly after completing the patent, I read in a book written for lactation consultants that there is not an artificial nipple on the market today that fills the baby's mouth the same way that his mother's breast does. I smiled to myself: Mine does!

I am currently working to make my new YUM Feeder available for market, for I believe it will be a cost-effective and genuinely helpful aid in nourishing cleft lip and palate newborns—both here in the States and wherever mothers don't have access to surgical options. Furthermore, it promises to reduce any threat of nipple confusion for even "normal" babies who might need to bottle feed or use a pacifier for any reason, for it replicates the fullness and softness of a mother's breast and nipple in the mouth.

It is my sincere hope that this booklet on breastfeeding will encourage mothers to persist in doing so—even when the process feels uncomfortable or discouraging. I've provided numerous "tidbits" of advice based on personal experience assisting thousands of newborns to breastfeed through the years. It is also my sincere desire to provide a more useful feeding device for those infants with special needs and/or sucking difficulties. My YUM Feeder is a simple and affordable solution for those thousands of newborns who can't readily breastfeed the natural way.

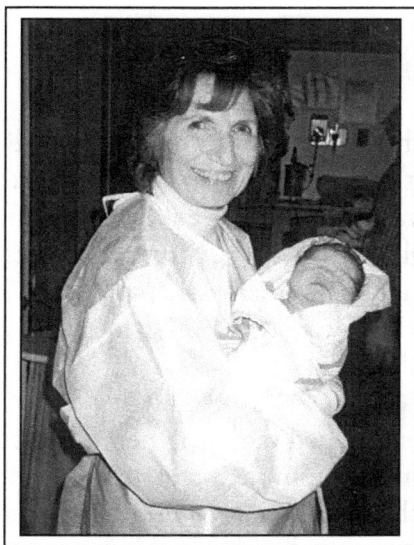

About the Author

Carolyn Gilmore is a retired Registered Nurse, Certified in Obstetrics. She graduated from nursing school in 1959 from Grace Hospital in Hutchinson, Kansas. In Wichita, Kansas, she worked in all areas of obstetrics and IV therapy before relocating to the Pacific Northwest in 1970. She spent a total of 41 years on night-shift, delivering babies and caring for newborns, serving her last 27 years at Newberg Community Hospital and then Providence Newberg.

During her lengthy and gratifying career, she assisted in approximately 2,200 deliveries and cared for nearly 17,000 newborns. In Newberg, she has had the privilege of caring for two generations of family members and enjoys spotting many of her now-grown-up "babies" around town.

Her passion for helping mothers to successfully breastfeed, as well as her own experience giving birth to a cleft lip and palate daughter who couldn't nurse in traditional ways, led Carolyn to design and patent a revolutionary new feeding device that will soon be available for purchase.

Testimonial

"As a nurse, I thought that if I prepared myself by reading books on breast-feeding, that it would be easy. Despite all my reading, I was still unprepared for how difficult it would be. Even though I was doing everything right, my baby didn't know what she was supposed to do. I was completely discouraged and ready to quit breast-feeding even though I knew 'breast is best.'

Carolyn Gilmore helped me using her 'Detour Method.' She made all the difference in my breast-feeding experince. Her method made things a lot easier, and her experience as an obstetrical nurse is invaluable. Carolyn is my hero! My baby is three months old now, and breast-feeding is a joy."

Sincerely,
Lisa

www.ingramcontent.com/pod-product-compliance
Lightning Source LLC
Chambersburg PA
CBHW070911280326
41934CB00008B/1680